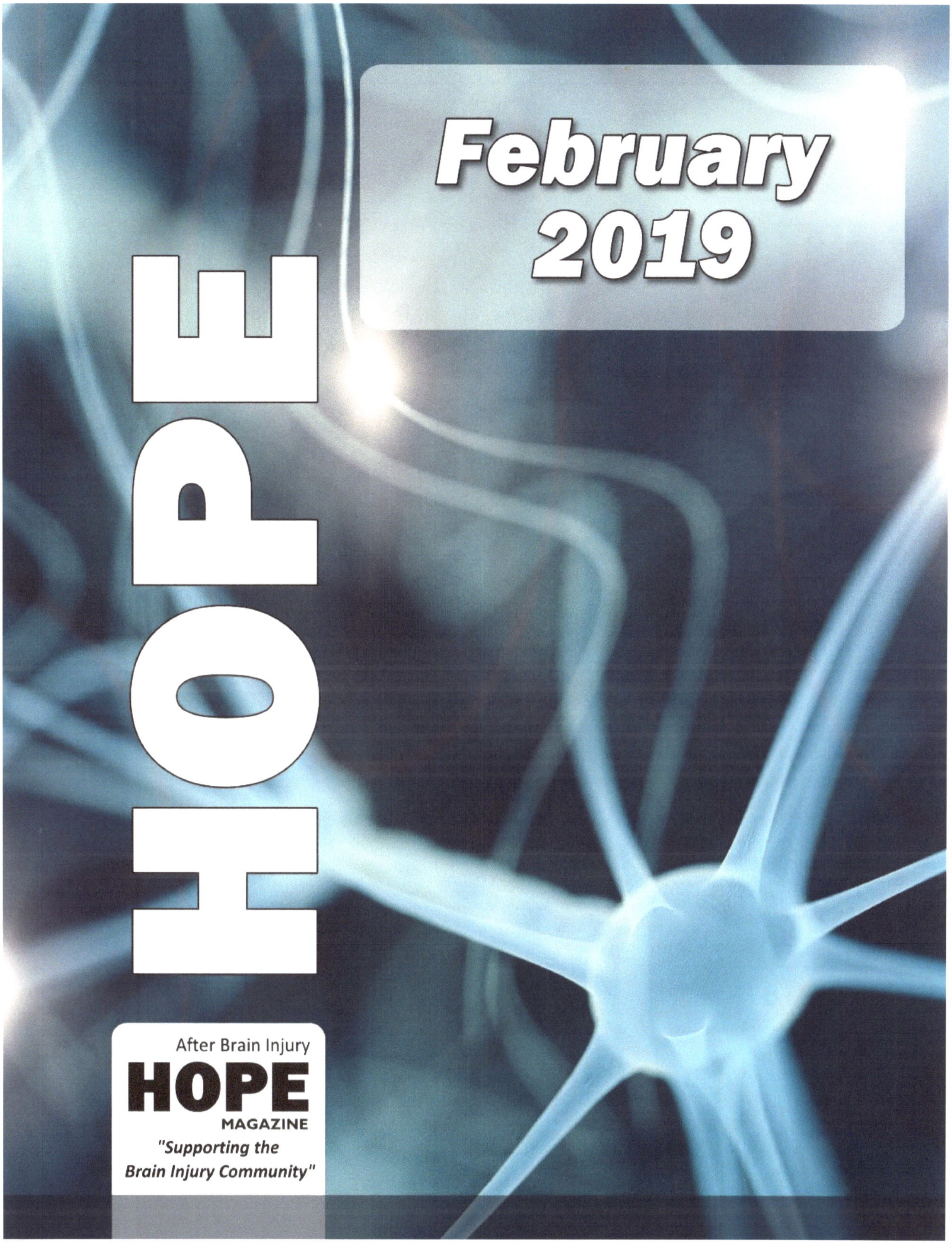

February 2019

HOPE

After Brain Injury

HOPE
MAGAZINE

*"Supporting the
Brain Injury Community"*

Welcome

HOPE MAGAZINE

Serving the Brain Injury Community

February 2019

Publisher
David A. Grant

Editor
Sarah Grant

Our Contributors

Mariëtte Loubser
Naomi Maendel
Jim Martin
Tracie Massie
Norma Myers
John Richards
Bridgid Ruden
Jeff Sebell
Loran Zumbrunn

Welcome to the February 2019 issue of HOPE Magazine

As we approach the four-year anniversary of our publication, it's hard not to be humbled. HOPE Magazine has grown from a few local readers to a worldwide publication read in close to sixty countries.

This month, we feature an issue that is truly international in scope, including contributors from as far away as South Africa and Australia. Brain injury is truly global in scope, but fortunately, so is brain injury recovery.

Together, as part of a worldwide support network, we lift each other higher and we support each other. One brain injury survivor at a time, we find the end to the isolation that many come to experience. We find hope!

It is my wish that you find something within the pages of this month's issue that help you along your journey.

Peace,

David A. Grant
Publisher

Contents

What's Inside
February 2019

> *Most of the important things in the world have been accomplished by people who have kept on trying when there seemed to be no hope at all.*
>
> -Dale Carnegie

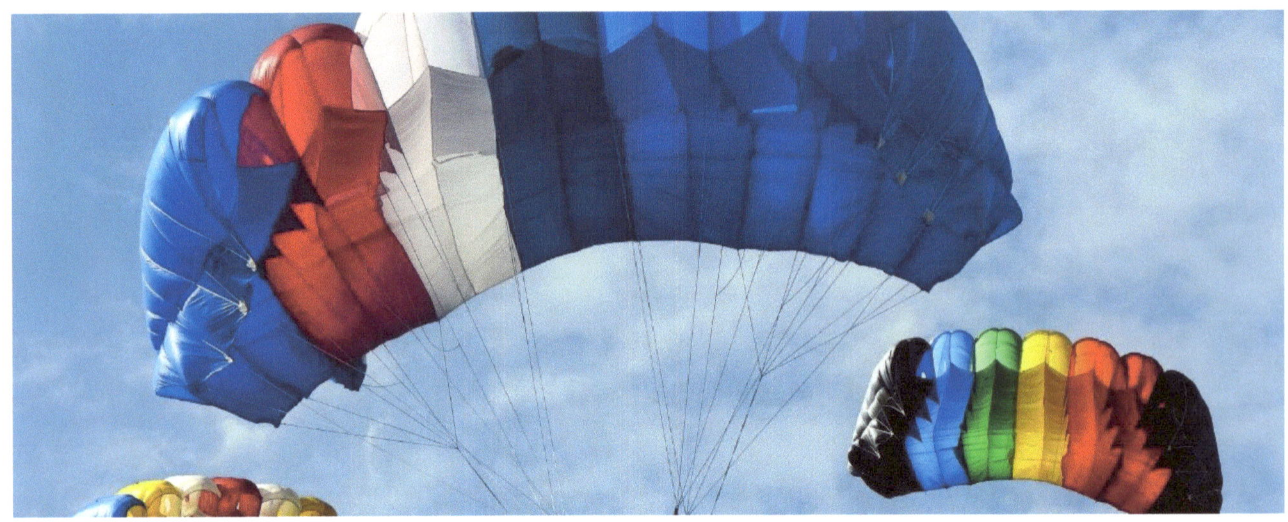

Skydiving Into a New Life
By Mariëtte Loubser

I am Mariëtte Loubser and my story is about miracles. In 2012, I started taking classes toward my master's degree in Inclusive Education. I was a high-school teacher and decided to do a tandem skydive for my twenty-fifth birthday. I found out that I just loved skydiving.

A school teacher by week, I was a skydiver on weekends. My first jump was perfect. On my second jump, disaster struck. It was February 23, 2013. Apparently, or so I am told, I started tumbling when I exited the plane. When my parachute opened, the line was blocking my parachute from opening completely. At the time, I was a student skydiver. They kept saying over the radio that I should pull my emergency cord. I was out and just hanging and never pulled my emergency cord. There were buildings next to the landing site. I fell on the rubble.

> "I never pulled my emergency cord. There were buildings next to the landing site. I fell on the rubble."

My family and club members waited for the ambulance. After examining me and assisting me, they said that I was too weak to be transported by ambulance. I was transported by helicopter to Milpark Hospital in Johannesburg, South Africa and arrived at 12:00 PM.

I broke many bones in my back including C1, T4, L4, L5, S2. I broke both my hips - the left one in two places, pelvis, coccyx, and tibia. I broke eight ribs, I tore my lung and sustained a severe traumatic brain injury, as well as a diffused injury. Since I was bleeding internally, I was too weak to be operated on.

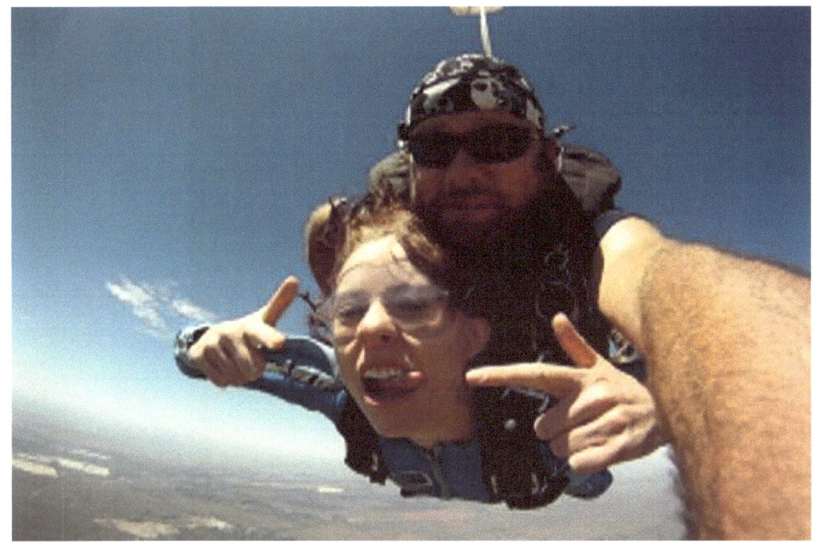

The head of the trauma unit was trying to stop the bleeding so that they could operate.

At twelve that night he said that I was on the verge of dying and that I could die because I was too weak. However, they needed to operate. I was in the operating room for three hours. They fixed my lung first, then added two plates to my ribs to repair them. After three-and-a-half weeks, I went to Netcare Auckland Park Rehabilitation Centre.

This was to be my home for the next three months. At the rehabilitation hospital, they had to re-teach me things that people take for granted as normal daily activities. My mother was there every day. She worked with me to improve my brain after I was at physio and occupational-speech therapy. My father and brother came to the hospital after work.

I don't remember ever skydiving, nor did I remember much of my teaching and master's program. In the beginning, I was angry at God. Why would he allow this to happen to me? My brain didn't register pain, so I didn't feel any pain in the beginning of my recovery. Later on, I started feeling the pain and I drank many painkillers that didn't actually take the pain away. Besides having pain due to my broken bones, I had a blocked tear gland in my right eye, constant dry eye and eye infections. I had double vision as well. Since my eye moved a lot, I could not get a prism in my glasses to eliminate the double vision.

I am a Type-A person and I started to remember more at the end of 2013. I resumed my master's program at the end of 2013 and began teaching in 2014, only after doing a trial lesson in 2013. Everything was such a struggle. It was like this until I realised that I needed to make the best out of the situation.

An article by Mike Strand in the November 2018 issue of HOPE Magazine puts it into words nicely:

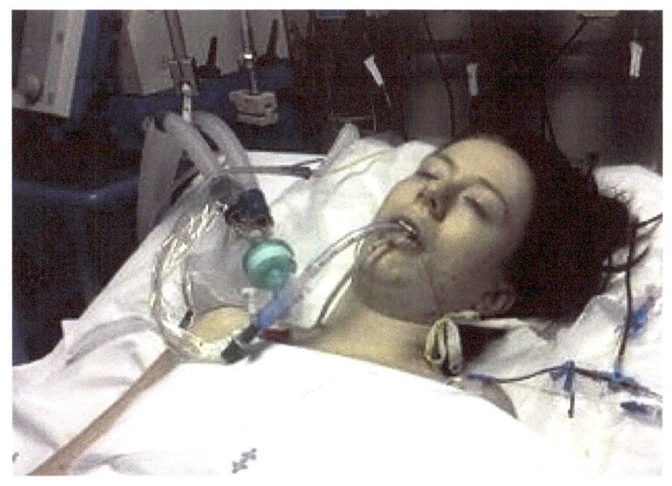

"Stephen Spender has put into words what it takes to succeed with peace and confidence while living with brain injury. I found it all too easy to bring myself down with unrealistic expectations. Trying to be the person I was before my brain injury was the chief unrealistic expectation that I had."

Things didn't change for me until I adopted a better attitude. It wasn't until I let go of trying to be who I was, that I began trying to be who I could be.

Thus, I decided to make the best of this unfortunate situation. I started joining many TBI groups on Facebook and Pinterest. I read books regarding brain injuries and got tips on how to cope with the situation. I also realized that no matter how much my accident and the after-effects frustrate me, there are people who have it worse.

What has helped me to cope is drinking lots of water to keep my brain hydrated. I read that seaweed helps brain injury. Now, I am drinking kelp tablets. I also read that essential oils help with brain fog and help in having a clear mind. I diffuse different oils to help me. There are days when I am going to have a day that I can't work due to headaches, aphasia or ongoing neuro-fatigue.

On these bad brain days I try to rest, but it is frustrating when I know I have work to do. What has helped me with this is to work ahead so that when I have these days, I don't have to worry about the work I need to do. I also write down everything as I have a poor memory. I put reminders on my phone to help with my memory.

Friends leave after brain injury. You see the true colors of people that say they care, love you and are your friends. My family and God have given me strength to carry on with each day. I finished my master's degree program in 2015. I wanted to give up many times, but my mother and father did not allow me to give up. I graduated in 2016.

I am Mariëtte Loubser from Johannesburg, South Africa and this is my story.

Meet Mariëtte Loubser

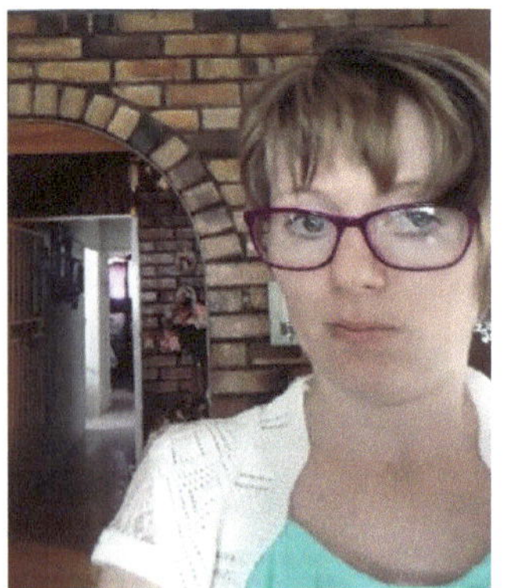

Mariëtte writes…

"I am Mariëtte Loubser from Johannesburg South Africa. Currently I am thirty-one years old, but when I had my accident, I was only twenty-five years old. I am currently a high school teacher. I finished my master's degree in 2015. I wanted to give up many times, but my mother and father did not allow me to give up. I graduated in 2016."

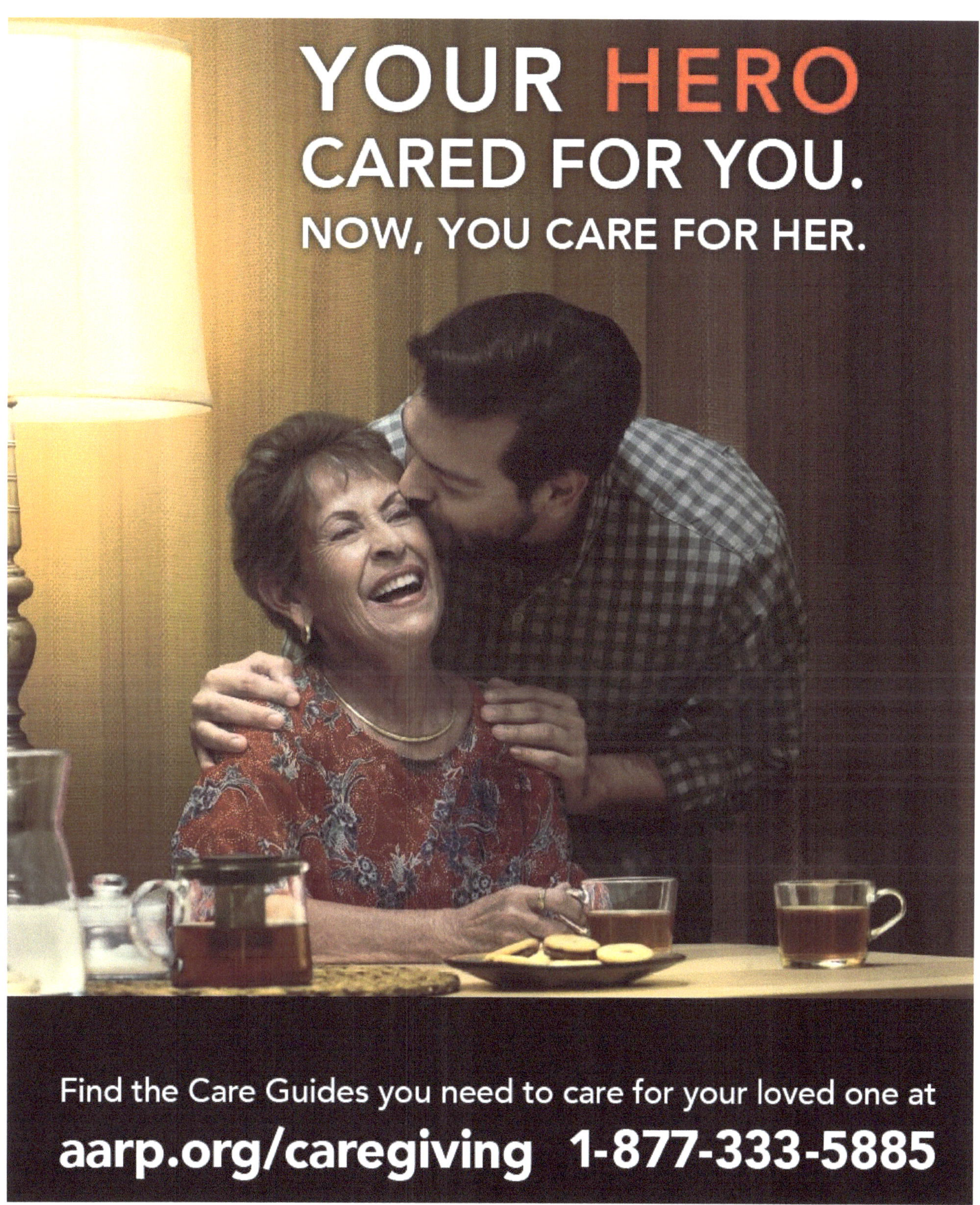

YOUR HERO
CARED FOR YOU.
NOW, YOU CARE FOR HER.
Find the Care Guides you need to care for your loved one at
aarp.org/caregiving   1-877-333-5885

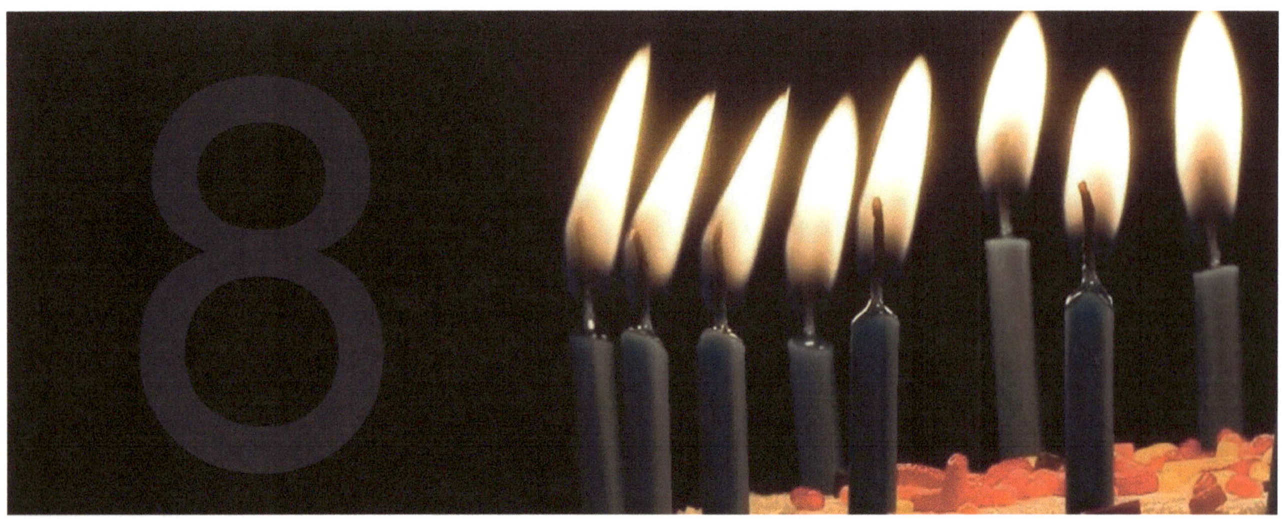

Eight Years Out

By Jim Martin

As I write this, it is eight years to the day when a good friend (who had a key to my home) found me unconscious at the bottom of a staircase. I suffered a traumatic brain injury and have no memory of the accident, nor the several weeks and months which followed. Recently, I obtained medical records from the three facilities in which I was admitted and treated following the accident. To say the least, reading these records gave me a new perspective on the significance of my injuries and, more importantly, how fortunate I was to survive.

For example, for the past eight years I was under the impression that I had been unconscious for approximately twenty hours. Yet, the initial

> "Since I do not recall the initial or specialty hospitalizations, I recently asked those close to me to describe their visits during that time period."

hospitalization reports that I had been "down" for up to forty-eight hours. Despite having suffered facial bone fractures, significant blood loss, and a crush/compartment syndrome injury to my left hand which led to rhabdomyolysis and acute kidney failure (breakdown of dead muscle proteins causing my kidneys to shut down), the TBI resulted in the most significant impairment.

Since I do not recall the initial or specialty hospitalizations, I recently asked those close to me to describe their visits during that time period. There were some funny stories, and some which were downright scary. For example, apparently, I insisted that Paul McCartney was in the building (one of the hospitals) and performed for the patients every Thursday! Where that came from, I have no idea. Apparently, I'm told, I had no sense of modesty and was quite disinhibited, as well as being unaware of my physical limitations. Much more problematic, several have told me that they were not sure if I would return - ouch, that hurt, but I'm sure I frightened them even more.

After being discharged from a fantastic rehabilitation hospital, for three months I lived in a foster care home which specialized in brain injuries. Even more frightening for me, is that after recovering physically, I thought I was ready to return home by myself and to my profession of thirty years, a successful trial lawyer.

I did not appreciate that I had a significant memory impairment, especially for new information, along with an inability to track conversations in groups of people. I received opinions from a treating neuropsychologist and physiatrist that I risked committing malpractice by trying to return to my profession. That was devastating. Then, the insurance company which was providing long-term benefits required I apply for Social Security Disability. I was lost. Dumbfounded. But, at the risk of losing the benefits, I applied, and on the initial application, it was accepted. And once my career was not available to me, so too, were many of what I thought were my good friends.

Of course, they had their families, careers and recreational activities which they continued to enjoy, as they should, but it left me to isolate.

Adding to my apathy was attempting to explain to new acquaintances why I was no longer practicing law, given my memory impairment, which was met with increasingly frequent comments such as "Well, you're sixty-ish, of course your memory isn't what it used to be..." Consequently, despite realizing that it was not healthy, I withdrew.

As more and more time has elapsed since experiencing my TBI and with the benefit of hindsight, I now realize that I struggled significantly during the first few years, to the point that I now believe that my overall recovery would have benefited by remaining at the foster care home for several more months.

It wasn't as though I could not function, alone as it were, but realistically I was somewhat emotionally incapable of grasping the significant changes in my life. I looked normal, I spoke well, I understood what was being said and what I read (although retaining that information was a vastly different matter).

I could no longer, realistically, define myself as a trial lawyer. I now see, again with the benefit of hindsight, that my life had become rather one-dimensional, which is never healthy.

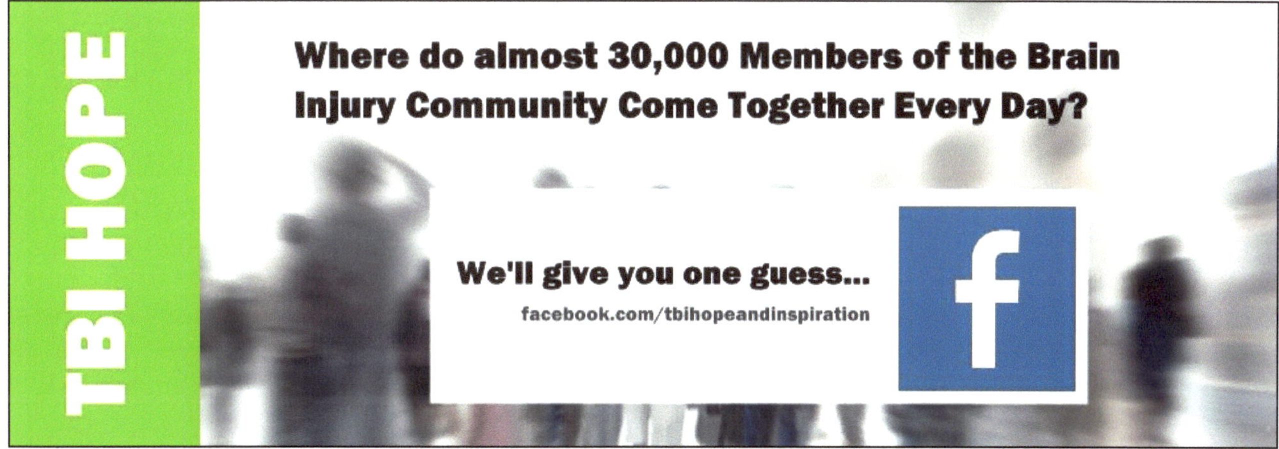

More recently, upon my questioning of the treating neuropsychologist and a subsequent consultation with a neurologist, I have been informed that in addition to being at risk for developing Alzheimer's, I am also at greater risk of developing Parkinson's and epilepsy.

As I confront these potential challenges, I have hope for the future that I will somehow be useful for the benefit of someone or something. What that may be, I do not yet know, but hope sustains me.

As I have previously written, the concept of hope is not easily defined for me. Dictionary definitions do not seem to suffice. Rather, the emotion which accompanies a sense of hope emanates from my heart, not my brain.

I realize that suggesting that I "think" with my heart may sound a bit crazy, but the more I learn from the research being performed by the HeartMath Institute, the more I believe that there is a significant connection between the head and heart.

And, I now consider the past eight years a transition. Sure, there were many significant changes, physical, professional, and personal, but the ability to keep moving forward is only possible with a sincere belief that hope, manifested through my heart, will lead me through this transition, the destination yet unknown.

Throughout my recovery, I have been drawn to the writings of Richard Rohr. Relatively recently, he posted comments and a quote attributed to Rabbi Harold Kushner which are extremely important for me.

"The greatest task for any person (brain injury or otherwise - my comment) is to find meaning in his or her life. Frankl saw three possible sources for meaning: in work (doing something significant), in love (caring for another person), and in courage during difficult times. Suffering in and of itself is meaningless; we give our suffering meaning by the way in which we respond to it."

Forces beyond your control can take away everything you possess except one thing: your freedom to choose how you will respond to the situation. You cannot control what happens to you in life, but you can always control what you will feel and do about what happens to you. This magazine, HOPE, has provided a venue for me to express the thoughts and feelings which have resulted throughout my recovery. For that, I am thankful.

Meet Jim Martin

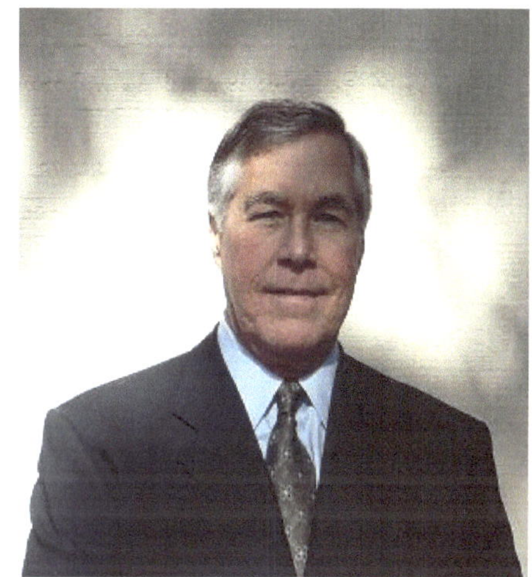

After 30 years practicing law as a trial attorney primarily representing physicians in medical malpractice litigation, Jim is a brain injury survivor whose career ended in December 2010 when he experienced a significant traumatic brain injury, and resulting permanent memory impairment.

Jim volunteers with the Alzheimer's Association, where he is a Board member, attends support group meetings with Brain Injury Connections NW, is a member of Brain Injury Alliance of Oregon, and volunteers at a local Portland, Oregon hospital.

To stay connected with the legal community, Jim mentors newly admitted lawyers with the Oregon State Bar.

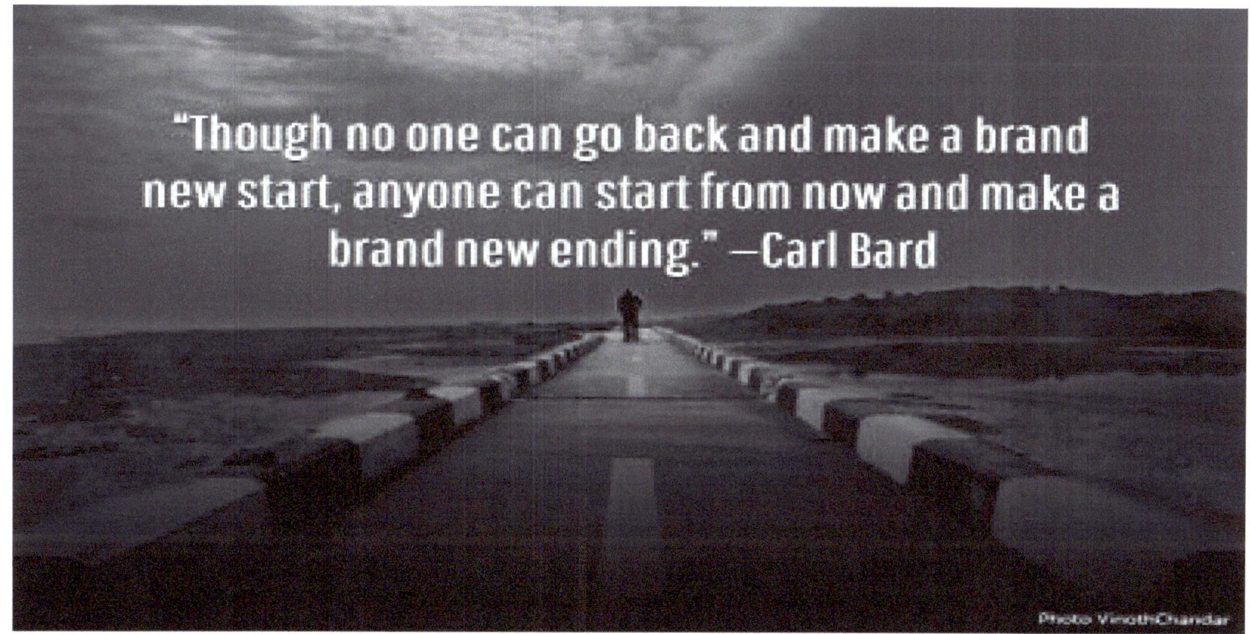

Ruby Red Slippers

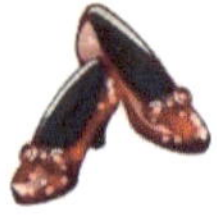

By Loran Zumbrunn

I used to enjoy Colorado to ski
It was a hobby where I really felt free
But luck ran dry and I got a bad dose
I hit my head and spent a week comatose

I suffered a traumatic brain injury
All my fight went into recovery
Prognosis was bad, but who gives a cluck ;)
Beat paralysis with stubbornness and luck

Three and a half months to learn to walk again
So determined, I'd climb any mountain
Support at Craig Hospital for so long
My family is ridiculously strong

Then here at Madonna I could always feel
Help everywhere, so my resolve was steel
I couldn't drive so I had to ride the bus
Rather freeze my toes than put up a fuss

Had a project at the Tractor Test Lab
It seemed to validate all of my rehab
Recovered for two years with no interfering
Before I attacked work in engineering

I was convinced this would just be a story
That I could break out to highlight my glory
I thought the old me would be back again soon
Until the hard truth gave me a new tune

At Kawasaki I achieved engineering
But soon I went from cheering to tearing
Worked long hours and gave all my energy
But I couldn't make up for my poor memory

They let me go and so far that I fell
Plenty of days I thought I was in hell

I was ashamed of my incapability
Making ends meet because of disability

I thought disability was pathetic
Until I needed to call the medic
I know my reasons are completely legit
But that doesn't mean I could stomach it

I thought about committing suicide
Decided no, mainly for family pride
That certainly won't help with depression
Passing days just to quell family's obsession

Motivational sayings I'd always receive
Things will get better, you've got to believe
I live on my own, so for that I am proud
At least while in front of a clapping crowd

We all have our own unique journey through s;)it
My compassion has multiplied because of it
I wish I'd have learned lessons with less pain
But growth regularly comes through severe strain

For me, a support group is nearly a must
A crowd who understands and I can trust
Empathy's great, but understanding is more
Acknowledging things normal people ignore

I've been forced to prematurely retire
Plus side is, my schedule earns people's ire
Deliberate effort for my world to recoup
I'm still searching for my new social group

After giving up hope to find a new career
I got one where I can bend the elders' ear
Grandparents get how my memory has cracks
But they see me push to fix where it lacks

I respect each person after my hassle
No longer looking down from my castle
A model human because of this drama
But that's only according to my mama

I don't know where all of the chips will land
But for now I have somewhere to happily stand
This could be viewed as a needed shake-up
But if I could click my heels, I'd love to wake up!

Loran Writes…

"Before my TBI, in 2014, I was a design engineer. I have written a poem about my life that I have shared with my TBI support group and it was received very warmly. They pointed out that having a brain injury can feel very lonely because people don't enjoy sharing the dark parts of their stories. I wrote most of my poem when I was in a very low place. I am willing, even excited, to share my personal story, especially if it can help others realize that they aren't the only ones feeling down, and progress can be made, even when it feels like you're in a bottomless pit."

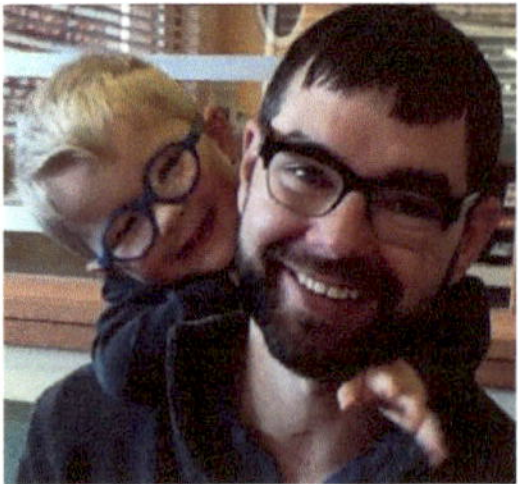

The Brain Injury Trap
By Jeff Sebell

I get a laugh when I mention to somebody that I lost my car in the parking lot and they respond with, "Oh yeah, I do that all the time."

I know they are just trying to be cute and funny or to find a way to make a connection with me, but what these people don't understand is that there is nothing cute or funny about a brain injured individual having to deal with constantly forgetting, misplacing or not understanding.

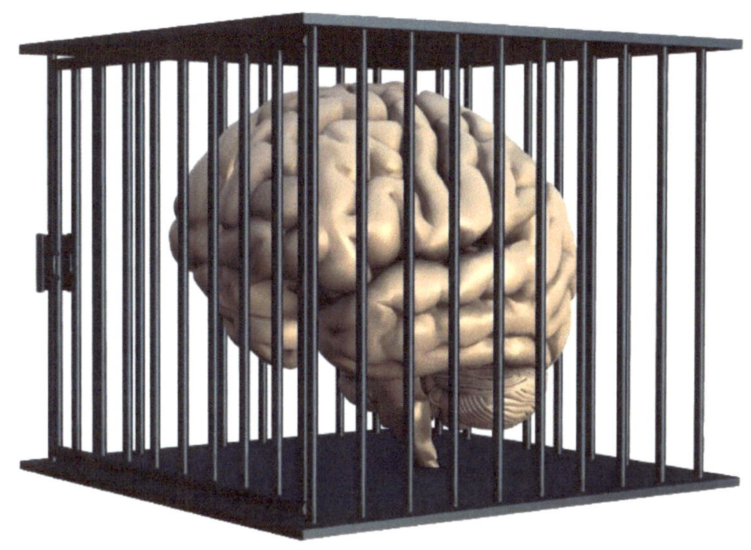

I'm sure many, if not all of you, understand exactly what comes with saying, "I lost my car again," when you have a brain injury.

You know about the confusion as you stand in the parking lot trying to remember where you parked, unable to figure out why you can't do something simple like remember where your car is. You know how that confusion gets worse, not better, the more you try and figure it out. You know about the frustration that comes with forgetting…yet again. You feel that not knowing where your car is parked is a reflection of what your life has become and that these type of things, which are just nuisances to other people, put you deeper and deeper into the abyss.

The last straw is that losing your car brings back every fear and frustration you've ever had, making you feel as though you don't belong on this earth.

I almost fell into that God-forsaken trap the other day.

Luckily for me, as I stood dumbfounded in the busy parking lot, teetering on the brink of the trap trying to suck me in, I had one of those rare revelations we sometimes have: you know, a flash of light and a single thought that cut through the fog and lit up the sky with clarity.

For that one great, shining moment, I saw the answer and I understood my life.

What was it that clicked?

In the millisecond just before I fell into the trap, I was able to pause and ask myself: What is really going on here? Why does it have to be like this?

It was in that moment that I took control.

Right then I understood that the "Brain Injury Trap" wasn't something that happened **to** me. The truth was this: I had brought the trap on myself. Yes, me. I didn't have the parking lot or the cars or my brain injury to blame, although that is very convenient. The trap was about to spring on me because I doubted myself, and the trap was like quicksand: the more I struggled and fought back, the harder it was to escape.

The Brain Injury Trap

In that moment I saw that I needed to do two things:

I needed to come to terms with the idea that due to my brain injury, I may sometimes forget where I park my car, and that's ok. That sort of thing will happen from time to time because I don't have a ton of control over how my memory works.

Secondly, coming to terms with this would help me accept "lil-ol' me" and stop me from beating myself up. It would also allow me to deal with situations constructively instead of using them as a reason to get mad at myself.

I saw that I needed to exercise control over my mind. Contrary to what I might think, it really wasn't the "forgetting" that was the issue. It wasn't the "forgetting" that made me a bad person. I made myself into a bad person by thinking I shouldn't be forgetting and by beating myself up and judging myself.

Making myself into a bad person springs the "Brain Injury Trap" on me.

Avoiding the Trap

So how do I avoid falling into the "Brain Injury Trap," the beat down I give myself, as well as the terrible lack of confidence I have, when I feel I can do nothing right?

We want to avoid the trap and reach the goal of having that shining moment of clarity and trust in ourselves, like I had the day I lost my car, last as long as possible. We must begin the process by accepting who we are. That will enable us to think objectively about the situation and we can move on from there, using our brains in a proactive and objective way.

> **"We must begin the process by accepting who we are."**

If I feel the trap coming on, I try to focus on things outside of myself. I try to turn myself into a *problem solver* rather than a *problem maker,* and the way I do this is by thinking about what I am *not* doing. I find that when I fall into the trap it is usually because I become very focused and create new problems by doing things over and over again and expecting things to be different; for example, I walk up and down the same aisle in the parking lot looking for my car because I think I must have walked by it.

These are the times I need to think expansively; think outside of myself so I can be more objective and not get caught up in doubting myself. Often the solution is very simple and I just have to give myself the room to find it.

Meet Jeff Sebell

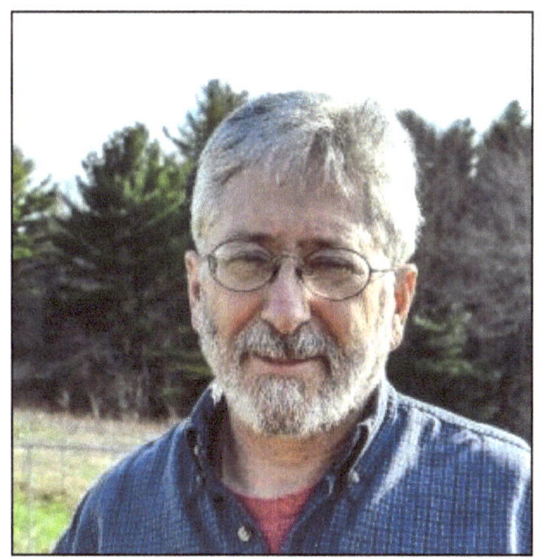

Jeff is a nationally published author, keynote speaker and blogger - writing about Traumatic Brain Injury and the impacts of his own TBI which he suffered in 1975 while attending Bowdoin College.

His book "Learning to Live with Yourself after Brain Injury," was released in August of 2014 by Lash Publishing. Jeff is a regular contributor to HOPE Magazine.

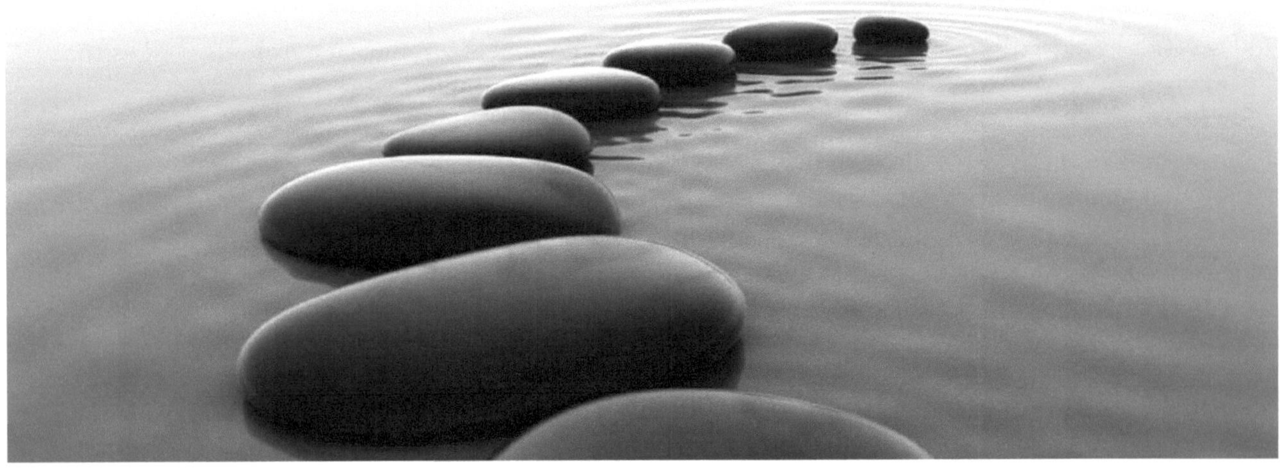

Caregiving Lessons and Confessions

By Norma Myers

After my son was diagnosed with a severe Traumatic Brain Injury in August 2012, despite the shock, I remember hearing Steven's healthcare providers repeating the word *caregiver*, over and over, as if they were determined to make me, of all unqualified people, claim the title. From the effects of double trauma, my own jarred brain could not grasp the reality that they were talking about me changing professions.

I could not understand why they were not checking the credentials of qualified professionals to fill this utmost important role of taking care of my only surviving son, Steven, if he woke up from his coma. I felt an urgency to scream that nowhere on my resume indicated that I was qualified to take care of a severely brain injured son. After all, how would I grieve the loss of my firstborn son, Aaron, (He did not survive the same accident that caused Steven's TBI) if I was expected to step in as caregiver to Steven. It all felt like a nightmare, one that I was more than ready to wake up from.

> "There's no candy-coating what happened after the knock on our door, delivering the worst news of our lives as parents."

There's no candy-coating what happened after the knock on our door, delivering the worst news of our lives as parents. Indeed, it was a nightmare! Aaron didn't survive the accident; Steven did sustain a severe TBI. My first confession was voiced to every professional that would listen: "Thank you for your vote of confidence, but I am NOT qualified to be Steven's caregiver!" The responses I received were not audible. Instead, I received sad smiles, pats on my shoulder, and head-shakes of despair from professionals at a loss for words.

Six years later, I can proudly say, without regret, I did step up. I changed professions. Being Steven's caregiver was the most rewarding professional title I have held. Another confession, it's not for the faint of heart, and payment is not in the monetary form. I honestly didn't think I had it in me, but I knew I had to do everything possible to get Steven through the most critical days of his life.

Caregiver lessons not embraced in the workforce:

- Quitting is not an option
- Deficits don't *define, they refine*
- A positive attitude changes your day
- It's okay to laugh at yourself
- Mistakes are fixable
- Take time to do a *little* something to make a *big* difference in the life of others
- Don't focus on the outside, respect the beauty on the inside
- Be kind, always
- Random acts of kindness should be a daily practice

The list of lessons goes on and on. I embrace each, while continuing to learn.

Due to Steven's fragile physical and emotional state, he did not learn of his brother's death until a month after the accident. I will never forget the dreaded day when I whispered those horrible words from my trembling lips into the ears of my fragile son. It was that moment, despite boot camp rehabilitation that Steven dedicated his recovery to his brother. Steven didn't give up, the fatal news made him fight harder. Through numerous major surgeries, blood, sweat, and tears, Steven kept his word to Aaron and made me proud to hold the prestigious title of his caregiver!

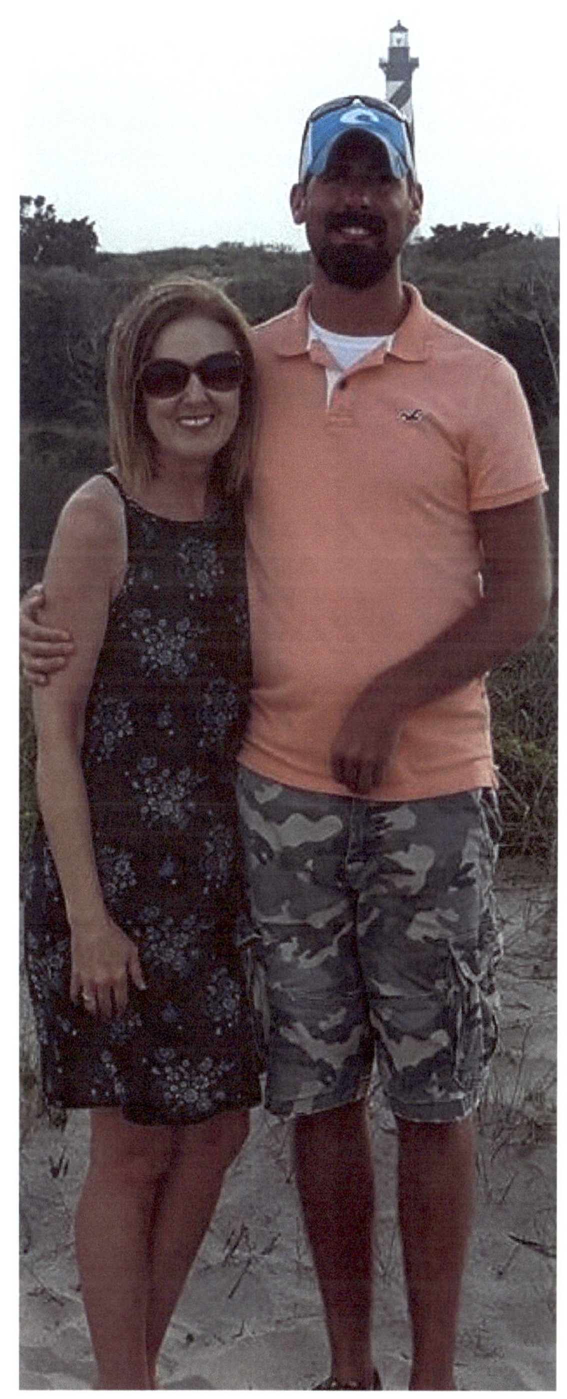

After experiencing caregiving up close and personally, I embrace the importance of being there for other caregivers. Caregiving is terrifying, exhausting and isolating. I was blessed to have a cooperative patient, devoted husband, supportive family, friends, and community. Not everyone has this, which is heartbreaking.

My list of confessions is longer than my allowed blog space, but in hopes of reminding other caregivers that you are not alone, here are a few highlights:

- My son's TBI struggles will be shared when appropriate, but his privacy will always be honored
- The caregiver manual sucks! Oh wait, you never received one, me either! That definitely sucks!
- It's okay, and a must, to ask for help
- You are not expected to know everything about caregiving. Tap into resources, they are out there, but you have to seek them out, no one knocks on your door with a caregiver's care package
- You can take a break, it's mandatory
- Don't hide your tears
- Don't feel guilty for laughing; it's medicine for the soul
- When asked if your smile is genuine, keep on smiling, it's so much better than a frown
- Exercise! A 30-minute walk is powerful
- Pray, meditate, whatever your belief, it's essential to your well-being
- Breathe! As in deep, to-the-core breathing
- Take time for yourself! This has been most challenging for me; I'm still working on it! We can't be present for those that need us if we neglect our own needs.

Most importantly, regardless of diagnosis, titles, or life situations, we can all agree that we live in a hurting and divided world. May we love respectfully and unconditionally. Instead of knee-deep ocean love, go all in, as in ocean bottom, exhilarating love, also known as the no-regret kind of love, which we all ultimately crave and need.

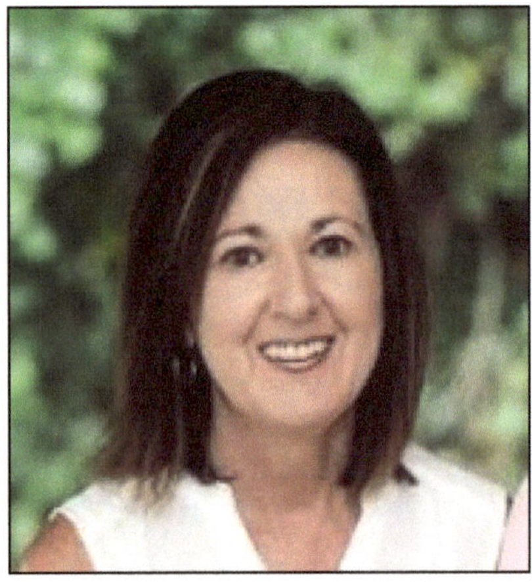

Meet Norma Myers

Norma and her husband Carlan spend much of their time supporting their son Steven as he continues on his road to recovery. Norma is an advocate for those recovering from traumatic brain injury.

Her written work has been featured on Brainline.org, a multi-media website that serves the brain injury community. Her family continues to heal.

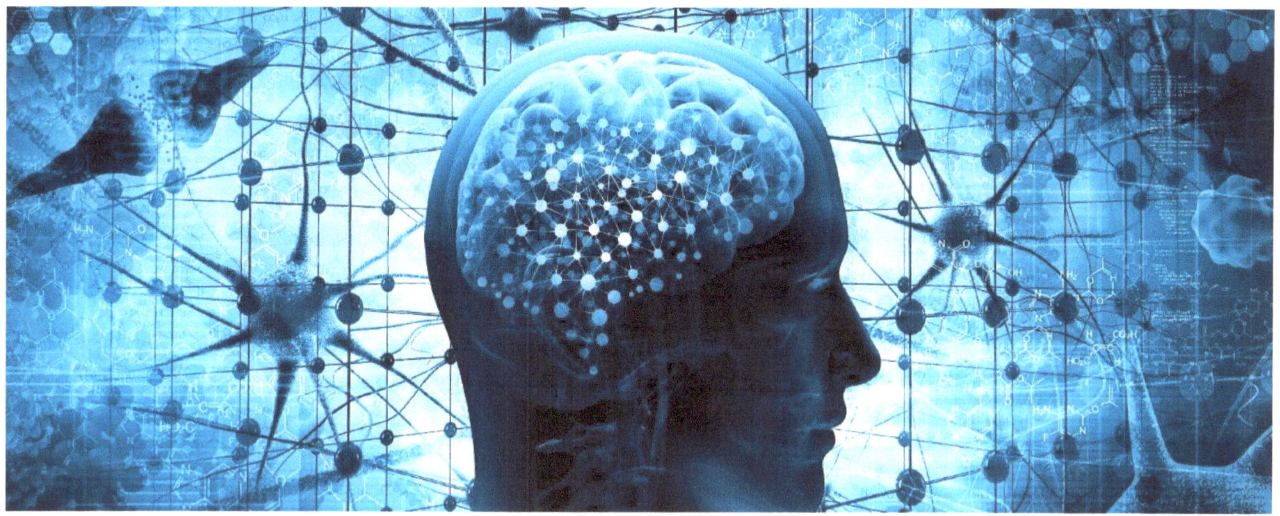

Simplistic Ways to Heal the Brain
By Bridgid Ruden

In May of 2008, a life-altering experience emerged in defiance of my life's vision. I was on a casual bike trail one morning with my girlfriend. A large degree of mud and water were present at the bottom of a hill. As I tried to pedal through this area, I lost control and smashed onto a hard, concrete surface, cracking my skull. I began bleeding from my right ear and nose, crying and screaming in pain. My CT revealed a brain damaged to the extent of having been in a car accident. I needed two emergent brain surgeries that day. My husband's concerns of my continual symptoms produced the necessity of a third brain surgery to remove a brain abscess. My final brain surgery, a titanium plate, was placed in my skull, as the previous one was infected. So many believed I would not survive, including a nurse who cared for me.

> "So many believed I would not survive, including a nurse who cared for me."

While in a coma, a spiritual clairvoyant woman shared that Archangel Raphael, Archangel Haniel and Archangel Metatron where with me, lovingly telling me I was dying. They were taking me to heaven. I shared with them that "I had a loving husband, three children and the continuous love I have for helping others to heal." They consulted God and decided that I could return to my life slowly but surely and I would need and receive incredible support. I struggled on life's roller coaster ride, yet I was supported and miraculously guided to become who I am today.

As I arose from my coma, I traveled back in time as a three-year-old, re-learning life's basic skills. With my disabilities, I was unable to return to my life as the mother and wife I was previously. Despite the odds, my husband never left me, as so many do. I had to let go of my meaningful career as an Advanced Registered Pediatric Nurse Practitioner. I cried so very often questioning, "God, why am I still here? What on earth is my life's purpose now?" Despite the incredible odds, I ventured forward to explore, develop and redefine myself. I learned how to move from suffering to healing; not just for myself but for so many others I encountered in mystical ways.

I began to identify the miraculous value of utilizing alternative health care to help heal my brain, body and spirit. I discovered the value of aerobic exercise. My physical therapist was stunned when I asked if I could jog toward the end of rehabilitation. Exercise creates new neurons in our brain which improves mental, physical and illness struggles. One year after my bicycle accident, I resumed riding the entire trail again on my own. I succeeded in completing the eleven-mile trail with tears of pure joy, as I resumed the trail where my brain had been severely traumatized. I was never going to quit riding a bike! I continue to exercise four to five days per week, focusing on both cardio and weight lifting. Talk about boosting my morale! It's a great way for me to begin my day.

The capability of nutritional healing enhances our brain healing and strengthens our immune and nervous system. My body was communicating a message to me when I began craving a diet high in dark green vegetables, salmon and fruit. Anti-oxidants diminish the impact of free radicals, which unfortunately impact body cells. Anti-oxidants are vegetables, fruit, whole grains, nuts and legumes. I continue to learn more about which foods support healing and which foods threaten my body.

It took me at least two years to truly laugh again. One of the incredible ways that I re-learned how to smile and chuckle manifested itself through laughter yoga! Of course, I never knew what laughter yoga was.

Powerfully, I was trained by an amazing brain injured survivor, who works at a rehabilitation center. Patients in rehab will pedal a wheel chair towards him and laugh hysterically! Laughter triggers the release of endorphins, which strengthens and rebuilds our immune system. Laughing ensures utter happiness, resolves stress overload, reduces pain and relaxes the whole body. Try coordinating this in your healing regime and witness what truly happens. Our brains need humor to grow.

Music therapy stimulates the entire nervous system and helps retrain the injured brain! It vitalizes and stimulates our vocabulary in amazing ways. Any brain-injured person with aphasia, who may only be able to say a word or two can miraculously sing an entire song! I have witnessed this several times and each time my mouth opens wide in amazement and joy. Wow! Visualize the power of music.

Dance is also very powerful. It enhances our thinking skills, motivation and memory. Dance provides a safe opportunity to reduce anger, frustration and depression. Despite memory loss, balance issues and vertigo, I shockingly remembered how to dance and play the piano. My brain was mesmerized by the power of music and body movement.

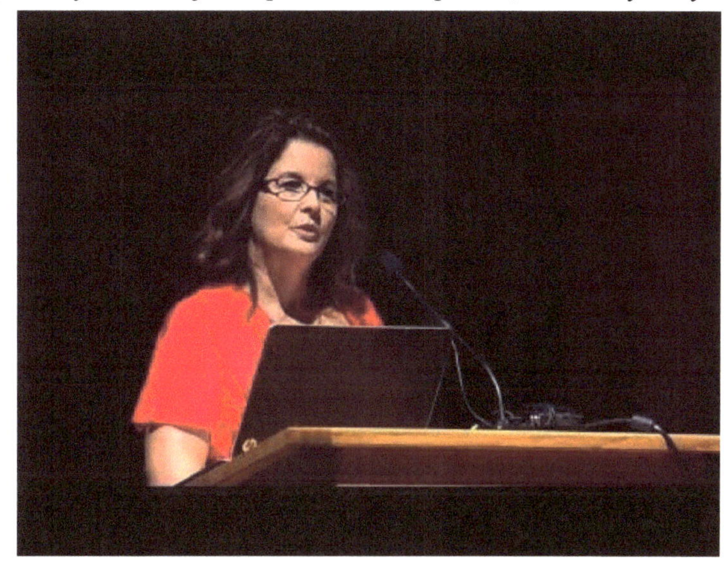

Bridgid Ruden Speaks About Traumatic Brain Injury

Despite my fear of not being an "artist," I explored art therapy. I was encouraged to attend a class by my friends with epilepsy. Our entire brain engages within art. Art guides the brain to heal from mental, emotional, and physiological impacts. Again, I was blown away by the simple ways to heal the traumatized brain. Medication doesn't solve all our body and brain's disabilities. It is only a tiny piece of true recovery.

In spite of my health care providers' and family's shock, I began reviewing my medical chart for answers about the trauma I endured and still denied. It was painful and shocking to discover what had occurred. With incredible Divine support, I bridged forward and created a PowerPoint presentation of my life's experience.

I was so challenged as I re-learned how to spell and create a sentence, and I could only read one-to-two pages slowly to understand. Shockingly, I proceeded to share my life's story to health care professionals and prior colleagues. Everyone, especially my speech therapist, was amazed. They had never seen a person with severe traumatic brain injury improve to the miraculous degree that I had.

When I share my life's miraculous adventure, people describe my presentation as: "Superb! It heals my soul." "A testament of what strength and determination can do!" "Moving speaker." Miracles continued to unfold in my life as I began successfully presenting my story both nationally and internationally and appeared on TV and radio stations!

The power of writing heals our brain in so many ways! I published articles and a chapter in a book, *Progression.* Unbelievably, I wrote my own book, *Discovering My Life's Purpose: From Tragedy to Triumph,* which is now an audio book.

My audio book has enlightened those with challenging disabilities as well as non-readers. My amazing sister Rachel is the narrator, since I continue to have aphasia. "Bridgid has the unique ability as an author to take the reader on this painful journey with her." "As Bridgid walks through each step of her rehabilitation, she inspired me through laughter, tears and her genuine spirit."

> ## "My audio book has enlightened those with challenging disabilities as well as non-readers."

I ventured forward to provide healing to those in need as a Reiki therapist, a spiritual healing artist. To give to others uplifts and blesses my spirit and continues to nourish my own healing.

No matter how much time has passed, when I'm introduced before I present my story, they share what I've accomplished. I am still in oblivion. I look around the room searching for her. "Who is she?" "I'd love to meet her!" I often hear, "She has found her calling!" Slowly, I am starting to understand that my life's purpose truly didn't leave me; it merely merged to a higher realm.

For all the miracles that I've been blessed with on my life's journey, I can't begin to say how grateful and honored I am to God and all the angelic people who lovingly guided and supported me in recovery. Never give up! Angels never leave us. I believe in you and always will!

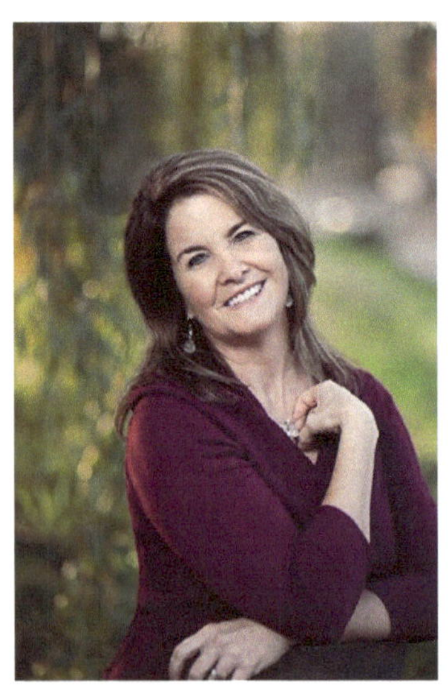

Meet Bridgid Ruden

In 2008, Bridgid suffered severe traumatic brain injury following a bicycle accident. Her life resumed as if she were a three-year-old as she went through the process of relearning even the most basic life skills.

Today Bridgid is an international keynote speaker and brain injury advocate. Her tireless work has helped countless others who have lives affected by brain injury. You can learn more about Bridgid on her website at www.bridgidruden.com. She continues to heal.

Introducing an Inspirational
New Book

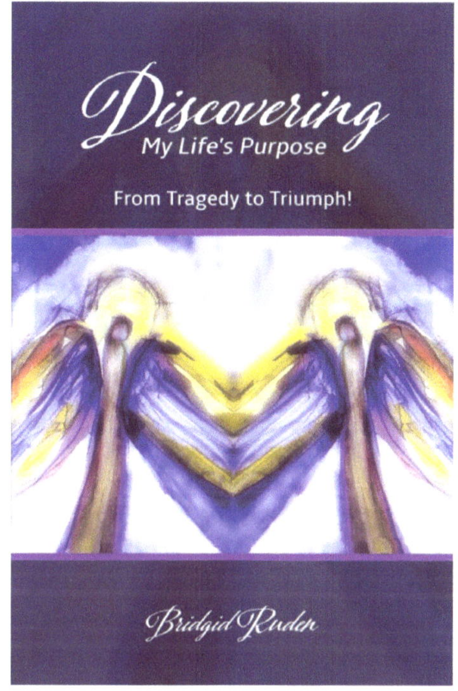

Now Available at

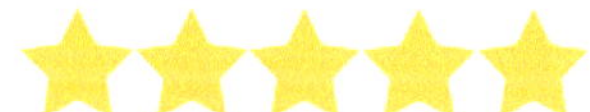

Discovering My Life's Purpose

From Tragedy to Triumph!

By Bridgid Ruden

★★★★★

The Five Star Reviews Are In

"Honest, beautiful writing! Bridgid has the unique ability as an author to take the reader on this painful journey with her."

"Incredible story of a brain injury survivor. Bridgid Ruden continues to be an inspiration as she shares her struggles and what has helped her in her healing journey."

"As soon as the book arrived, I started reading it & couldn't put it down. Bridgid has a beautiful way with her words & her flowing style of writing makes ones feel like you're sitting in front of her listening to her."

Meet Bridgid Ruden

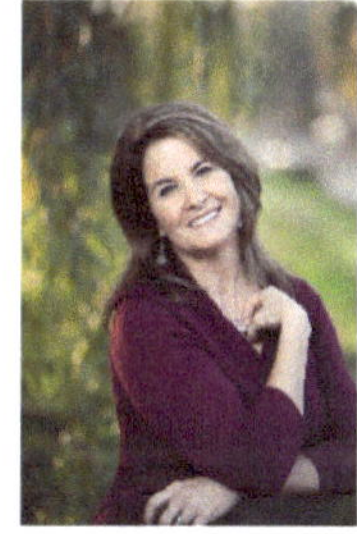

As she awoke from a coma from severe traumatic brain injury, she re-emerged into life as a three year old, slowly re-learning how to utilize her startled brain. Unbelievably, she miraculously ventured forward as she began to share her life's story both nationally and internationally as a keynote speaker.

www.bridgidruden.com

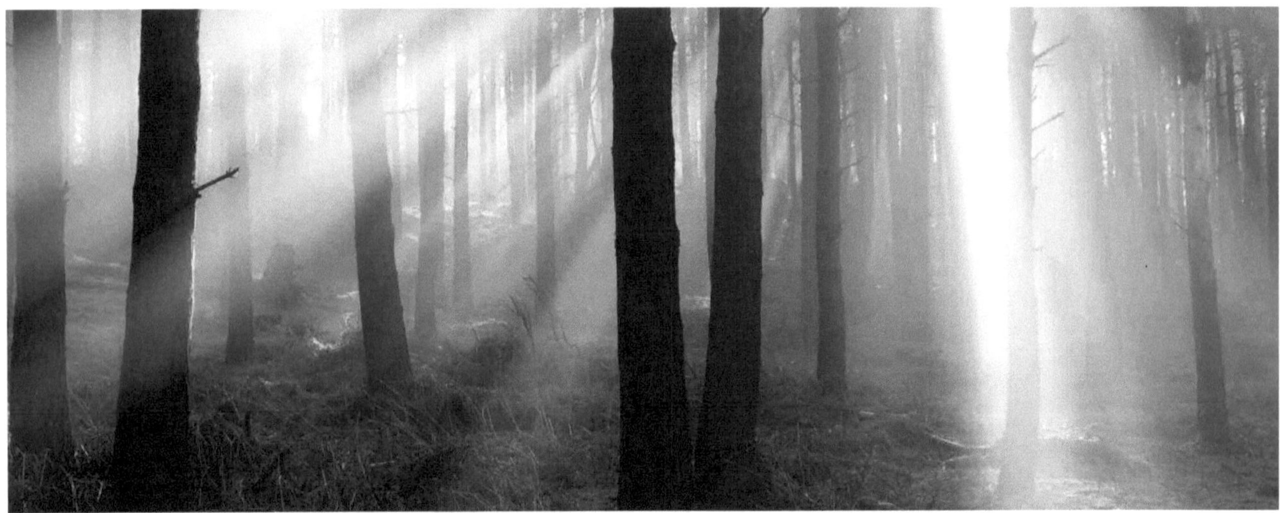

After the Fog Clears
By Tracie Massie

Where to start? After nine weeks in the hospital, "The Fog Cleared" (which is what my son said it felt like after the final stages of waking up from his coma). It had been an agonizing year of non-stop doctor appointments and my son was graduating from high school. I foolishly thought our lives would settle down.

I noticed the problem during the summer of his senior year. He would have outbursts of anger and get upset but they only lasted a few minutes and were gone. Things started getting progressively worse and his physical medicine doctor sent us to psychiatrist who specialized in children and teenagers with TBI. He started my son on a new medication and it worked miracles! He wasn't back to "normal" but I was slowly realizing this was our "new normal."

> "I noticed the problem during the summer of his senior year. He would have outbursts of anger and get upset but they only lasted a few minutes and were gone."

In the midst of all of this, he became a father. I have a beautiful granddaughter who is now eight years old. Things were tolerable for a while. He was still difficult to deal with at times, but I could always calm him down. Around the summer of 2014, he rented a house. I managed the money, but he did great! He had a cousin move in with him who helped to keep him settled down and focused, so things were pretty good. He lived in the house for three months but had to move when the landlord sold the property. What seemed like a good move wasn't so good after all.

His new home was in walking distance of a grocery store, three pizza places, his pharmacy and unfortunately, the liquor store. It seemed great at the time because he didn't have a driver's license, so it helped me a lot. Unfortunately, he started drinking more and more. He was up to a pint of whiskey a day and several beers. If that wasn't bad enough, he became friends with the neighbor, and it seemed like something wasn't right. I told my son that I thought the neighbor was selling drugs, but he wouldn't listen.

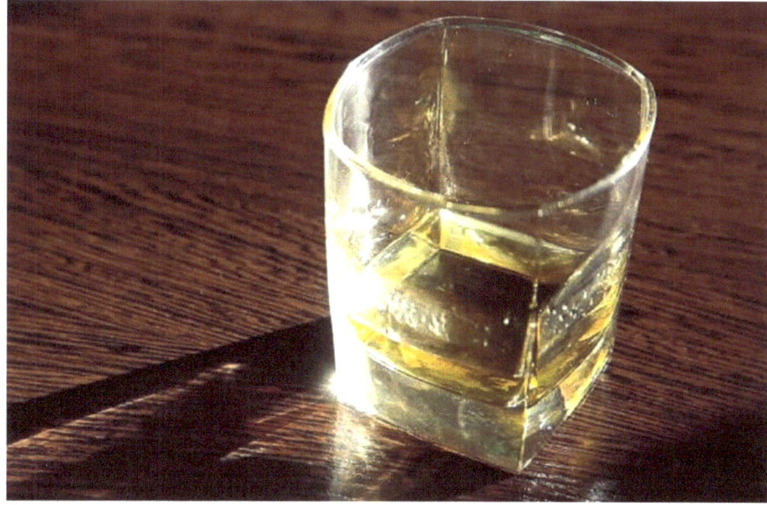

One evening there was a knock at his door by a uniformed police officer and one in a SWAT uniform. They told him that the man I was suspicious of was stepping out my son's back door and selling drugs! They did say that they knew my son wasn't involved but if they came back to his house again, they wouldn't be knocking on the door. Needless to say, the friendship ended. During his stay at that address he received two petty theft charges, received another TBI from three guys jumping him, and he got married.

My son and his wife managed to find an apartment in a small town about ten miles from where he lived and I thought it would be great – same problem, different place. He also developed a bad habit of letting people stay with him for extended periods of time. Unfortunately, these people made no contribution to the household so it fell back on me.

Through all of this everything seemed to fall in my lap. If he was mad, I was the one the anger was aimed towards. My physical and mental health were deteriorating. It seemed as though every day brought several new problems. He would call me continuously wanting something. If I ignored the calls, he called every family member looking for me. One weekend from Friday evening to Sunday evening, I had over two-hundred phone calls from him. He was belligerent with me. He threatened me.

Finally, after one more apartment I managed to find him a house, closer to me and cheaper rent. There have been ups and downs here also, but lately he seems to be calming down and not so angry towards me. When he has these spells, it can be scary to someone on the outside, but I know there is enough of the young man I raised inside him, that he would never hurt me. He has cut his drinking back to one or two beers a day and I'll take that. In a perfect world, he wouldn't be drinking at all, but it's not a perfect world. I know it sounds like I'm complaining but I'm not. I feel very blessed that he survived the accident and is as independent as he is. Believe it or not, I haven't touched the tip of the iceberg with the events of the last thirteen years, but I don't want him to seem like a monster, because he's not. He gets so frustrated with the way he acts sometimes but he continues to try. That October day in 2006, my son walked out the door. My laid back, soft hearted, gentle son walked out. Nine weeks later I brought him home a very agitated, angry, sarcastic young man. He sees the change in himself too. We all mourn the loss of the young man that his step-father and I raised but we are here to help him in his struggle to exist in a world that doesn't understand. He has no friends from school because I don't think they know how to take him. He jokes and people take him seriously because of his expression not changing. Fortunately, he has a friend and a cousin that stick with him regardless, and I am very grateful for them.

He has improved a lot with medication changes, changes in his environment and I have been running off the free-loaders. I just pray I will have a day of peace and quiet soon.

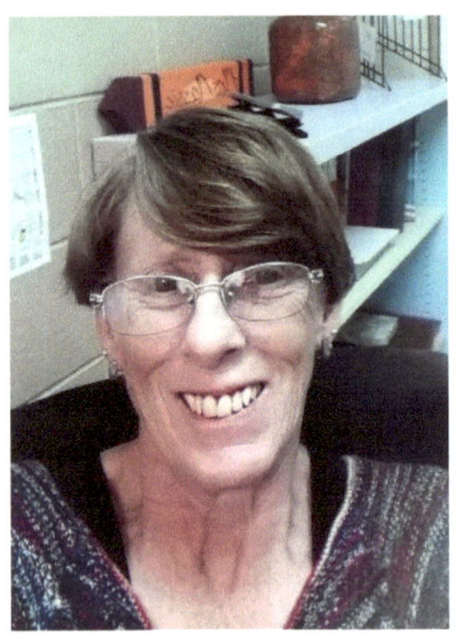

Meet Tracie Massie

Tracie writes…

"I live in Darbyville, Ohio and work for our local school as a teacher's aide for special needs and IEP students. I am the mother of a TBI survivor. My son's first TBI occurred when he pulled out in front of a semi in 2006. He has suffered two more TBI's since. I wrote this to let other caregivers know they are not alone."

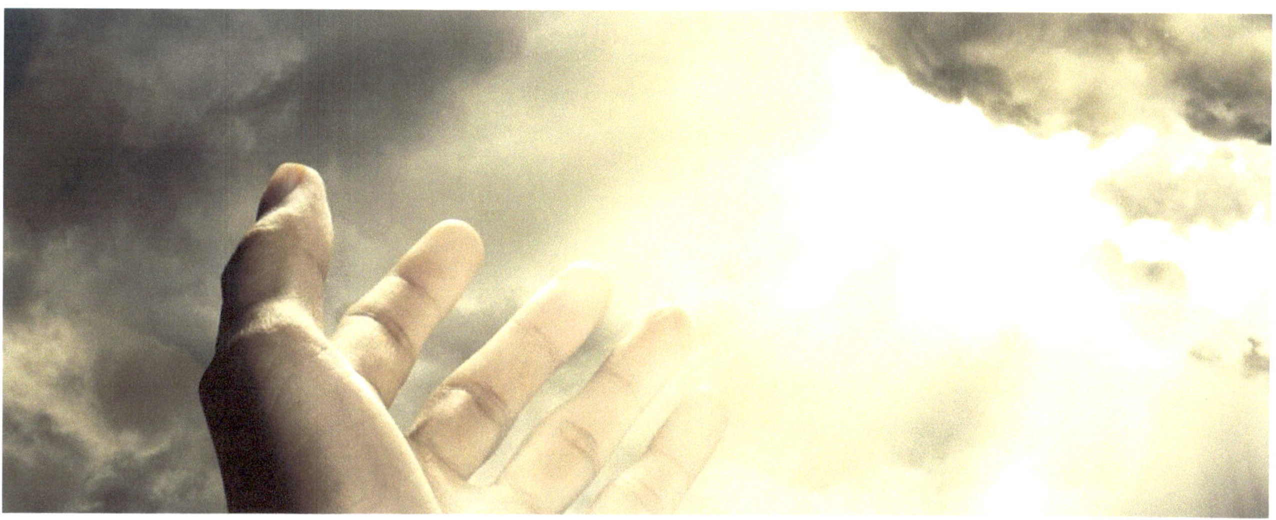

It's Not Easy Being a Miracle
By Naomi Maendel

On May 14, 2017 I suffered a subarachnoid hemorrhage – a ruptured brain aneurysm. It came with no warning and I had none of the risk factors. I had endovascular coiling surgery two days later. There were complications and I was put into a coma for sixteen days to bring the pressure in my brain under control. Overall, I spent a month in hospital – I don't remember most of it. I spent another month in a rehabilitation center, rebuilding my basic cognitive functions, balance, and strength.

From the beginning I showed a remarkable lack of physical or cognitive damage. My double-vision and unsteadiness on my feet gradually disappeared. The crushing fatigue improved. Mentally, I could remember, comprehend, and communicate as before. I was slow and it took a lot of energy, but it was there from the start. It took time to rebuild basic things like standing, walking and reading, but it came within a couple months. People were surprised at how normal I seemed and how functional I was. I returned to my job six months post-surgery, working part time; in a little over a year, I was back at full time. People often call me a miracle and I believe I am.

> "It took time to rebuild basic things like standing, walking and reading, but it came within a couple months."

This story isn't really about that.

Before my aneurysm, I struggled with an anxiety disorder for nearly ten years. During my time in hospital and rehab I felt great calm and great peace. I felt very loved and supported by my family and church. I thought the peace would last. I thought my near-death experience had put all my anxieties in perspective – they seemed very small. I had come through a great trial and handled it well. It seemed that the days of anxiety were over for me. God had brought me through something awful in order to change my perspective and heal my anxiety, and now I would be all better.

Boy was I wrong. It turns out there aren't any shortcuts, not even for miracles. Instead of putting out the fires of anxiety, my brain injury added napalm. The real struggle began when I returned home from rehab. The exhaustion, feeling left behind by healthy family and friends who had resumed their lives and the emotional strain of a life suddenly altered, began to wear me down. I struggled with panic, fear, depression, guilt, and loneliness like never before. My own mind became a very unsafe place with dark, confused thoughts I couldn't control or pull out of.

I couldn't turn to the distractions of work or friends or entertainment for long because my injured brain could only handle short periods of communicating, colors, and sounds. Being overstimulated and exhausted only heightened everything I felt. By the six-month mark I was desperate to return to work, to escape from my mind.

With the help of God, my family, a good therapist, a caring and patient church family, my faith, my dog, medication, and time, I'm slowly emerging from that hole. I still struggle with it, especially when I feel fatigue, which happens regularly. The challenges of mental illness and brain injury are very similar. There's no timeline or pattern of recovery, no rulebook or map to lean on when the self-doubt hits. Since both are unseen, we look normal, making it easy for people to underestimate, minimize, or deny the struggle it truly is.

I've found one of the greatest challenges to be the responsibility it places on me; since mental illness and brain injury can't be fully seen or measured, my medical treatment relies heavily on my ability to communicate with

"My own mind became a very unsafe place with dark, confused thoughts I couldn't control or pull out of."

professionals – their ability to ask questions and listen, and my ability to describe my experiences fully and honestly.

This demands a lot of trust, and even more, the courage to be honest with myself. This doesn't develop overnight, and not without missing opportunities and making mistakes.

I also struggle with being a miracle. My daily challenges are so small compared to other ABI and TBI sufferers. Shouldn't that make me feel more grateful, more at peace, more positive? I fight with myself when I feel frustrated, disappointed, fearful, and doubtful. The ups and downs, the instability, is hard to take even though it's a road of improvement. People still tell me I'm a miracle and I still agree, but I'm still a real person who struggles. People don't want to hear that; they want a simple, quick, happy ending. I run up against their disappointed expectations all the time and I hope in time it'll bother me less.

I'm slowly giving myself permission to struggle, to feel how I feel. What I've learned is that being grateful isn't a feeling; it's a framework, an orientation. So being grateful can include everything we feel, even emotions that we think don't fit. Some days it's easy, other days it's a minute by minute battle. I'm happy to say that the easy times are slowly getting longer.

I'm grateful for Brain Injury HOPE Magazine and the other survivors who share their stories. They make me feel part of a community of extraordinary people. Their honesty helps me be honest. Their strength in the midst of weakness and struggling gives me strength. Their company makes me feel less alone. Their tenacity, heart, hope, and courage take my breath away. They help me accept myself where I am and look forward to better days, receiving and giving encouragement along the way.

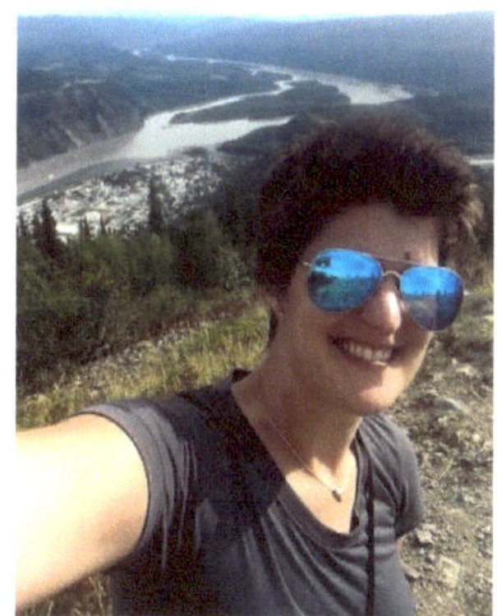

Meet Naomi Maendel

Naomi Maendel is a library technician who lives in Winnipeg, Canada. She enjoys cooking, cycling, cross-country skiing, singing in choirs, and playing with her dog Bentley.

Reaching for the Positives
By John Richards

Sustaining an illness or injury can be a difficult, lonely, unpleasant experience that lasts much longer than anyone thinks it should or wishes it would. Further, one person may "get the diagnosis" but a significant illness or injury is more of a family affair, impacting spouses, children, parents and the whole family.

Now let's be clear from the start: Having a brain injury really stinks, and please be aware that this is a family publication and that much more could be said about the experience of brain injury that cannot be printed here. You know what I mean.

Further, nothing is going to be in this article that is going to represent a quick or easy or simple cure. There is no such thing when it comes to brain injury. This article is about looking at the positives as a strategy and a lifestyle to achieve the best possible outcomes and life going forward, given what you have to deal with.

> "This article is about looking at the positives as a strategy and a lifestyle to achieve the best possible outcomes and life going forward, given what you have to deal with."

There is an entire branch of study called positive psychology, which endeavors to look at strategies and methods to assist us all to become more positive and also that looking towards gratitude and optimism offers tremendous benefits and health improvements as life goes forward.

To give you an example of exactly how difficult it is to move your thinking toward the positives: back in September of 2001, I was lying in a bed at the Northeast Rehab Hospital in Salem, New Hampshire, when a gentleman I had known for some time through the Brain Injury Association came to visit me.

He sat on the end of my bed as people do in hospital visits and we talked for a bit. He then said to me that he thought that his brain injury was one of the best things that ever happened to him.

I was in the hospital and couldn't walk. I was eating through one of those tubes, out of work, and had to live in the rehab every day. I was a total mess. I immediately assumed that he was totally crazy, that his brain injury had addled his brain, and that the best thing I could try to do was to escape from the hospital – an idea that did not work so well.

He went on to explain that he had a very different life after his injury. Previously he had been nonstop, flying all over the country and hardly seeing his wife and children. However, after his injury he was able to be more present with all of them and able to engage in many more enjoyable activities. He was not being so pressured all the time and just generally enjoying life a whole lot more.

And now, many years later, I am not sure that I totally agree with him regarding brain injury being the best thing ever, but I certainly do agree that looking at the positives has made it a whole lot better.

It has paid off for both him and for me. Let's look at some effective strategies for positivity: meditation, daily gratitude, and self-compassion.

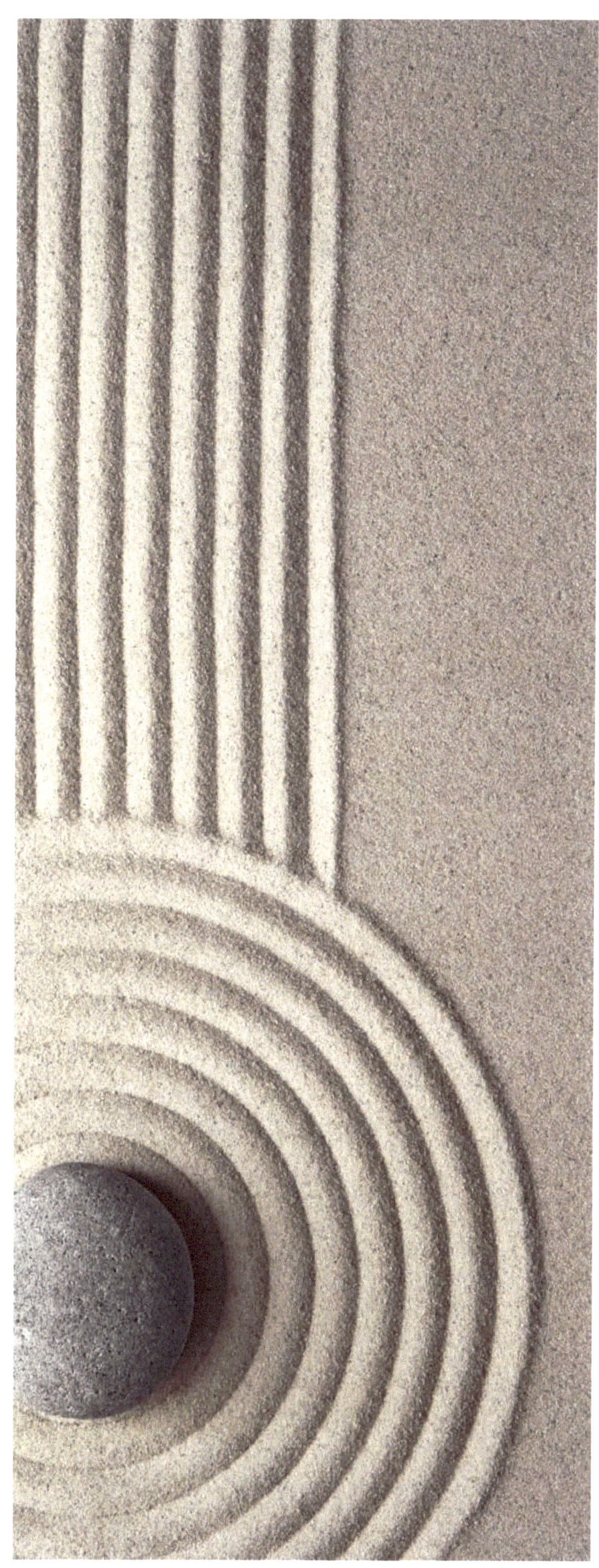

Meditation. There are lots and lots of ways to meditate. But most important is not to find a perfect form of meditation — it's to form the daily habit of meditation.

Commit to just two minutes a day. Start simply if you want the habit to stick. You can do it for five minutes if you feel good about it, but all you're committing to is two minutes each day.

Pick a time and trigger. Not an exact time of day, but a general time, like morning when you wake up or during your lunch hour. The trigger should be something you already do regularly, like drink your first cup of coffee, brush your teeth, have lunch, or arrive home from work.

Find a quiet spot. Sometimes early morning is best, before others in your house might be awake and making lots of noise. Others might find a spot in a park or on the beach or some other soothing setting. It really doesn't matter where — as long as you can sit without being bothered for a few minutes. A few people walking by your park bench is fine.

Sit comfortably. Don't fuss too much about how you sit, what you wear, what you sit on, etc. I personally like to sit on a pillow on the floor, with my back leaning against a wall, because I'm very inflexible.

Others who can sit cross-legged comfortably might do that instead. Still others can sit on a chair or couch if sitting on the floor is uncomfortable. Zen practitioners often use a zafu, a round cushion filled with kapok or buckwheat. Don't go out and buy one if you don't already have one. Any cushion or pillow will do, and some people can sit on a bare floor comfortably.

Focus on your breath. As you breathe in, follow your breath in through your nostrils, then into your throat, then into your lungs and belly. Sit straight, keep your eyes open but looking at the ground and with a soft focus. If you want to close your eyes, that's fine. As you breathe out, follow your breath out back into the world. If it helps, count: 1. breathe in, 2. breathe out, 3. breathe in, 4. breathe out.

When you get to ten, start over. If you lose track, start over. If you find your mind wandering (and you will), just pay attention to your mind wandering, then bring it gently back to your breath. Repeat this process for the few minutes you meditate. You won't be very good at it at first, most likely, but you'll get better with practice.

And that's it. It's a very simple practice, but you want to do it for two minutes, every day, after the same trigger each day. Do this for a month and you'll have a daily meditation habit.

Develop Your Gratitude Journal

Every day, before you go to bed, take at least five minutes to remember the positive emotions that you savored during the day, and on the weekend take ten-to-fifteen minutes to look at all the positive emotions of the past seven days.

How did you feel this week compared to other weeks? Are there any differences? How do you feel right now?

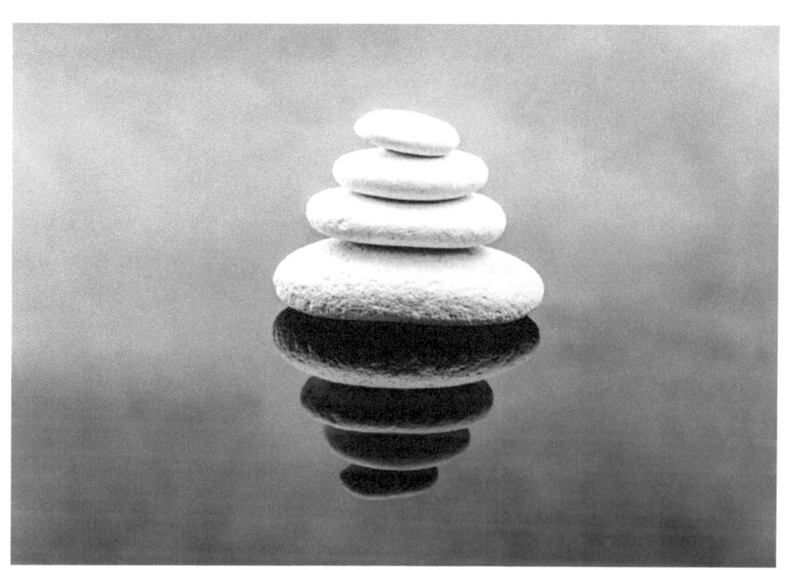

Practice every day before going to sleep by making sure to list at least three things you are grateful for today. They do not have to be grand or profound: you will not win megabucks every day. What are you thankful for? Did you enjoy the dinner that your caregivers made for you today? Did you appreciate that someone made it? Did you enjoy a special event? Were you glad for warmth and sunshine?

People who practice daily gratitude wind up with much more enjoy happiness in life.

A Letter of Self-Compassion to a Wonderful, Loved Person

Have you ever heard of self-compassion? Simply put, self-compassion means that you treat yourself with care and concern when confronted with your own mistakes, failures, and shortcomings. It has three different components: Self-kindness, a sense of common humanity, and mindfulness.

This specific exercise is called *A Letter of Self-Compassion.*

Imagine someone who is unconditionally loving, accepting, and supportive. This friend sees your strengths and opportunities for growth, including the negative aspects about you. The friend accepts and forgives, embracing you kindly just as you are.

Now write a letter to yourself from the perspective of this kind friend. What does he or she say to you? How does this friend encourage and support you in taking steps to change? Let the words flow and don't stress about structure or phrasing.

After fully drafting the letter, put it aside for fifteen minutes. Then return to the letter and reread it. Let the words sink in. Feel the encouragement, support, compassion, and acceptance. Review the letter whenever you are feeling down about this aspect and remember that accepting yourself is the first step to change.

"Patience is the calm acceptance that things can happen in a different order than the one you have in mind." (ref: PositivePsychologyProgram.com)

I have found that by looking at the positives as a strategy and a way of life, my life as a brain injury survivor has improved immensely. If it works for me, it can work for you – but only if you are willing to try.

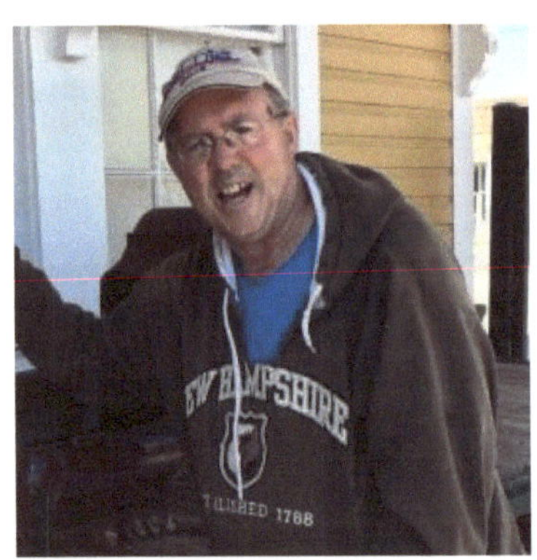

Meet John Richards

John Richards is a stroke survivor currently living in Peterborough, New Hampshire. John is the former president of the Brain Injury Association of New Hampshire's board of directors and a current board member. He is also a member of the New Hampshire Governor's Commission on Disability. He's known by those close to him for an occasional epic road trip.

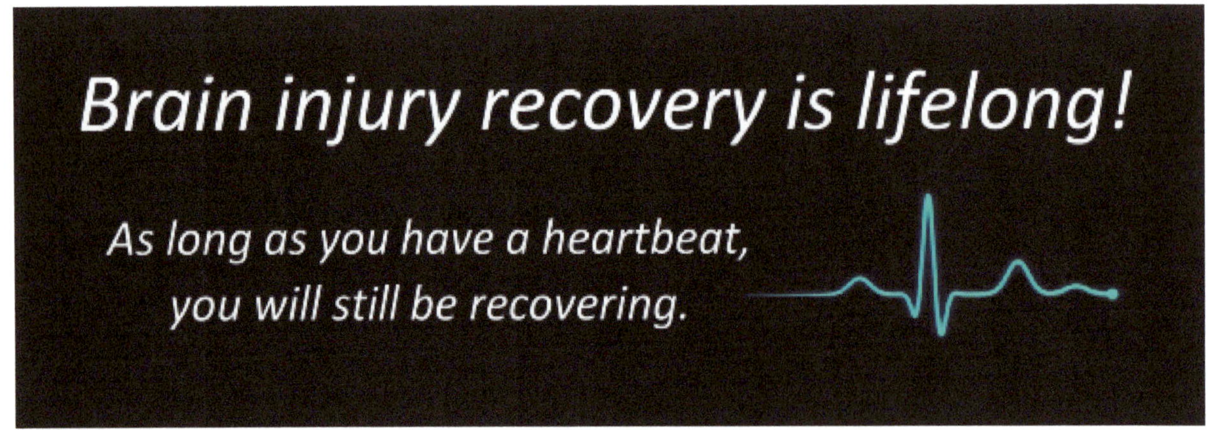

News & Views

We think that you'd agree that this is a pretty amazing issue of HOPE Magazine. Early on, after brain injury became part of our lives, in our naiveté we thought that all brain injuries were *traumatic brain injuries.* As we grew in the type of knowledge and understanding that comes only with time, it became quite clear to us that there were many living with brain injuries that were not traumatic.

From stroke survivors, to those living with anoxic brain injury, and more, we learned that we needed to be more diverse in the stories that we feature in our monthly publication. This month set the bar for diversity featuring stories by stroke survivors, TBI survivors, as well as family members.

From Canada to New South Wales, to our United States contributors, we are delighted to share stories of real hope and inspiration from around the globe. Brain injury does not discriminate, nor is it mindful of borders. Every twenty-one seconds someone sustains a brain injury – making the numbers add up quickly. In less time than it took to read this month's issue, almost fifty people experienced a brain injury.

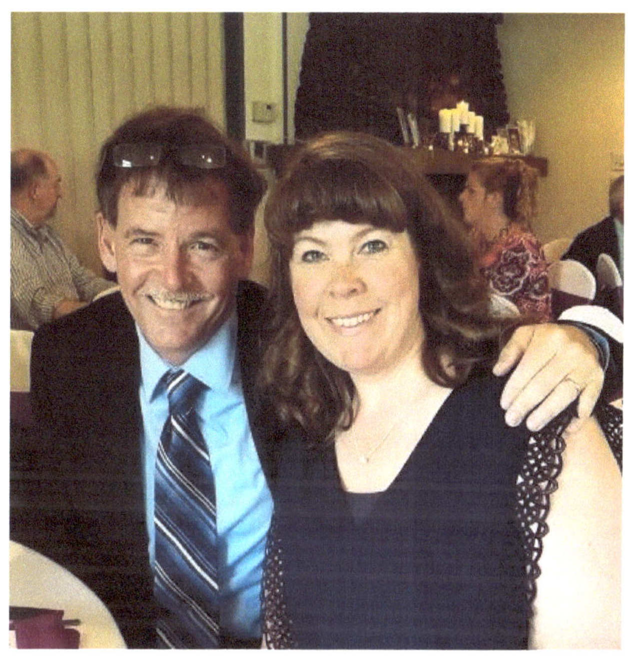

It is our continued hope that we can serve not only the current brain injury community, but future survivors and their families.

Next month is Brain Injury Awareness Month. Watch for our upcoming special March issue!

Peace.

~David and Sarah